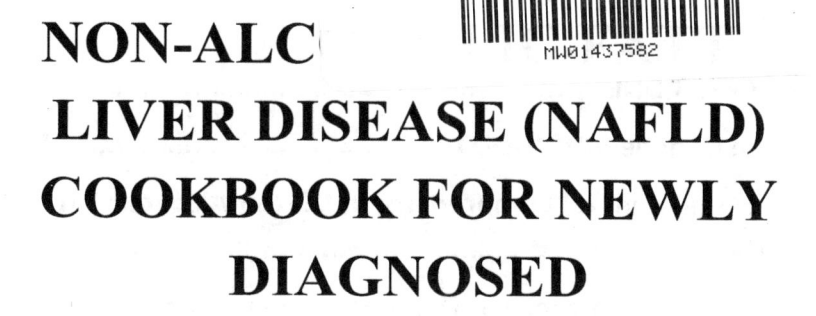

NON-ALCOHOLIC LIVER DISEASE (NAFLD) COOKBOOK FOR NEWLY DIAGNOSED

Nutritious Recipes, Lifestyle Tips, Meal Plans, Medical Insights, And Strategies To Combat NAFLD And Promote Liver Wellness

DR. ERIC TRISTAN

CONTENTS

CHAPTER ONE 10
  An Overview Of NAFLD 10
  A Fundamental Comprehension Of Non-Alcoholic Fatty Liver Disease 11
  Dietary Importance In The Management Of NAFLD....12
  Guidelines For Dietary Support For NAFLD 15

CHAPTER TWO 18
  A Balanced Plate Contributes To Liver Health 18
  Consuming Lean Proteins As Part Of Your Diet 20
  Vital Fats To Promote Liver Health 23
  Making Intelligent Choices Regarding Carbohydrates And Fiber 26
  The Significance Of Vitamins And Minerals In Liver Health 29

CHAPTER THREE 32
  The Effects Of Hydration On NAFLD: An Emphasis In The NAFLD Cookbook.. 32
  Methods Of Meal Planning For NAFLD: 34
  Recipes For Delectable And Liver-Friendly Breakfasts:37
  Ideas For Nutrient-Dense Lunches For NAFLD 38

CHAPTER FOUR 42
  Appetizing Dishes To Promote Liver Health: 42
  Snack Alternatives That Promote Liver Function 45

- A Variation On Desserts: Delightful Treats For NAFLD ... 47
- Liquids Influencing Liver Health 49

CHAPTER FIVE 52
- Practices Of Mindful Eating For NAFLD: 52
- A Comprehension Of Portion Control 54
- A Knowledge Of NAFLD-Compatible Cooking Methods 56
- Integrating Physical Activity Into One's Daily Routine 57
- Techniques For Managing Stress To Promote Liver Health 59

CHAPTER SIX 62
- Guidelines For Eating Away With NAFLD 62
- Progress Monitoring And Commemorating Achievements 66
- Frequent Concerns Regarding NAFLD And Diet 70
- Conclusion 74

THE END 77

Copyright © 2024, By Dr. Eric Tristan

All Rights Reserved

All rights reserved. No part of this book may be reproduced, distributed, or transmitted in any form or by any means, including photocopying, recording, or other electronic or mechanical methods, without the prior written permission of the author, except in the case of brief quotations embodied in critical reviews and certain other noncommercial uses permitted by copyright law.

DISCLAIMER

The information provided in this book, is intended for informational purposes only. The content is not intended to be a substitute for professional medical advice, diagnosis, or treatment. Always seek the advice of your physician or other qualified health provider with any questions you may have regarding a medical condition. Never disregard professional medical advice or delay in seeking it because of something you have read in this book.

The author of this book has made reasonable efforts to ensure that the information provided is accurate and up-to-date at the time of publication. However, the author makes no representations or warranties of any kind, express or implied, about the completeness, accuracy, reliability, suitability, or availability of the information contained within these pages.

Any reliance you place on the information provided in this book is strictly at your own risk. The author shall not be liable for any loss, injury, or damage arising from the use of this book or the information contained herein.

The mention or reference to any individuals, products, websites, organizations, or other names within this book does not imply endorsement by the author. The inclusion of such references is solely for informational purposes and does not constitute an endorsement or recommendation.

Furthermore, the author disclaims any association or affiliation with any individuals, products, websites, organizations, or other names mentioned in this book.

It is important to consult with a qualified healthcare professional before making any dietary or lifestyle changes, especially if you have a medical condition. Each individual's health situation is unique, and what works for one person may not work for another.

Again, the information provided in this book is not intended to diagnose, treat, cure, or prevent any disease or health condition. Always seek the advice of a physician or other qualified health provider regarding any medical questions or concerns you may have.

Thank you for your understanding and for taking the necessary precautions when considering the information presented in this book.

ABOUT THIS BOOK

This book entitled "Non-Alcoholic Fatty Liver Disease (NAFLD) Cookbook" tackles a substantial health concern that impacts a considerable segment of the global population. NAFLD, a common liver condition distinguished by hepatic fat accumulation, is frequently associated with sedentary lifestyles and poor dietary habits. This cookbook is an invaluable resource for individuals who have been diagnosed with non-alcoholic fatty liver disease (NAFLD) or are interested in its prevention. It offers exhaustive guidance on nutrition and meal planning strategies that are specifically designed to promote liver health.

The significance of this book resides in its capacity to enlighten readers regarding NAFLD and enable them to formulate well-informed dietary decisions. By acquiring a fundamental comprehension of the disease and the significance of diet in its control, individuals can adopt a proactive stance to enhance their liver health and general state of being. This book emphasizes the importance of maintaining proper hydration and adopting mindful eating practices, in addition to the significance of including lean proteins, healthy lipids, and carbohydrates abundant in fiber in one's diet.

An essential element of this book is its comprehensive compilation of delectable and nutritious recipes. This cookbook provides a wide variety of meal ideas that promote liver function, including nutrient-dense breakfasts, scrumptious dinners, and even inventive pastries. Furthermore, it offers recommendations on how to incorporate portion control, mindful eating, and stress management strategies—all of which are integral elements of a comprehensive approach to NAFLD management.

Additionally, this book responds to frequent inquiries and concerns regarding NAFLD and diet, providing pragmatic recommendations for dining out and monitoring advancements toward health objectives. Additionally, it underscores the significance of integrating physical activity into one's daily routine, as exercise is indispensable for enhancing liver function and metabolic health as a whole.

In conclusion, this "Non-Alcoholic Fatty Liver Disease (NAFLD) Cookbook" serves as a highly beneficial resource for individuals impacted by NAFLD or those with an interest in enhancing liver health via dietary and lifestyle adjustments. This book equips readers with practical guidance and evidence-based information, enabling them to assume agency over their health and implement beneficial modifications that can significantly endure and improve their overall well-being.

CHAPTER ONE

An Overview Of NAFLD

Non-alcoholic fatty liver disease (NAFLD) is a highly prevalent chronic liver condition that affects individuals on a global scale. Non-alcoholic fatty liver disease (NAFLD), denoted by the buildup of adipose tissue in the liver cells, frequently affects individuals who abstain from excessive alcohol consumption, hence the nomenclature "non-alcoholic." This disease comprises a spectrum of manifestations, including non-alcoholic steatohepatitis (NASH), a severe form of liver damage that can advance to cirrhosis and liver cancer.

Individuals who have risk factors including obesity, type 2 diabetes, insulin resistance, metabolic syndrome, and elevated cholesterol levels are more prone to developing NAFLD. A sedentary way of life and unhealthful dietary selections serve to worsen the condition. NAFLD, despite its widespread recognition, frequently manifests no symptoms during its initial phases, posing a diagnostic challenge in the absence of specialized testing.

A Fundamental Comprehension Of Non-Alcoholic Fatty Liver Disease

Among its many vital functions are nutrient storage, detoxification, and metabolism. An overabundance of calories, especially those derived from toxic lipids and carbohydrates, induces the liver to accumulate surplus energy in the form of fat. As time passes, the accumulation of excess fat may surpass the hepatic organ's capacity, resulting in cellular injury, inflammation, and oxidative stress. These mechanisms are implicated in the advancement of NAFLD and its associated complications.

In addition to inflammation and damaged liver cells, additional factors contribute to the progression from simple obese liver to NASH. NASH is associated with an increased risk of fibrosis progression, which can culminate in cirrhosis and liver failure. Furthermore, NASH is associated with an elevated risk of cardiovascular disease, demonstrating the systemic ramifications of NAFLD that extend beyond the hepatic organ.

NAFLD is diagnosed through the utilization of diverse imaging modalities, including computed tomography (CT), magnetic resonance imaging (MRI), and ultrasound. Blood and liver function tests may also detect irregularities in lipid profiles and liver enzymes, which would necessitate additional investigation.

Dietary Importance In The Management Of NAFLD

Dietary intervention is an essential component in the treatment of NAFLD. The condition frequently emerges as a consequence of lifestyle factors, including unhealthful dietary selections, lack of physical activity, and obesity. A cookbook for those with NAFLD emphasizes the significance of consuming a nutritious, well-balanced diet that is nutrient-dense while minimizing caloric intake and hazardous dietary components.

Typical NAFLD-friendly dietary components include:

1. Adherence to a Diet Low in Processed and Saccharine Foods: An overindulgence in processed foods, refined carbohydrates, and saccharine beverages can worsen the accumulation of liver fat and insulin resistance. The cookbook advocates for the replacement of these ingredients with fruits, vegetables, and whole grains as a means to support liver function and stabilize blood sugar levels.

2. The consumption of healthful fats, including avocados, almonds, seeds, and olive oil, has been associated with potential benefits for individuals with NAFLD, including inflammation reduction and improved lipid profiles. While emphasizing these healthy lipids, the cookbook restricts the use of saturated and trans fats, which are prevalent in fried foods and meaty meats.

3. Balanced Macronutrients: For the management of NAFLD, it is vital to consume a balanced amount of carbohydrates, proteins, and lipids. The cookbook offers recommendations regarding portion sizes and advocates for the intake of unsaturated lipids, lean proteins, and complex carbohydrates to enhance metabolic health and satiety.

4. Consume nutrient-dense foods: Low-glycemic fruits, verdant greens, cruciferous vegetables, and lean proteins are examples of nutrient-dense foods. These foods are abundant in vitamins, minerals, and antioxidants, which aid in the detoxification pathways of the liver and mitigate oxidative stress. The cookbook emphasizes these ingredients in a variety of flavorful and satisfying recipes.

By following the dietary guidelines provided in the NAFLD cookbook, individuals can proactively enhance liver function, decrease the accumulation of liver fat, and lessen the likelihood of disease advancement.

Guidelines For Dietary Support For NAFLD

The nutritional recommendations outlined in the NAFLD cookbook function as a strategic guide for individuals aiming to enhance their dietary practices and efficiently cope with their condition. Important recommendations comprise:

1. The implementation of mindful eating and portion control practices can effectively discourage the overconsumption of calories and facilitate weight management, both of which are essential components in the management of NAFLD.

2. Adherence to Moderation in Added Sugar Consumption: Prudently restricting the consumption of sweetened beverages and added sugars can effectively regulate blood glucose levels and mitigate the likelihood of developing insulin resistance, a characteristic feature that is characteristic of NAFLD.

3. Enhanced Intake of Dietary Fiber: In addition to supporting weight loss efforts, dietary fiber regulates blood sugar levels and promotes gastrointestinal health. The cookbook advocates for the ingestion of foods that are abundant in fiber, including whole cereals, legumes, fruits, and vegetables, to enhance digestive function and facilitate satiety.

4. Sufficient hydration is a critical factor in maintaining optimal liver function and overall well-being. It is advised by the cookbook to drink plenty of water and botanical infusions while limiting consumption of caffeinated and saccharine beverages.

5. Tailored Approach: Acknowledging the potential for individual variations in dietary requirements, the cookbook promotes the adoption of a personalized nutrition strategy. Seeking guidance from a registered dietitian or healthcare professional can assist in customizing dietary recommendations to accommodate unique dietary restrictions, cultural inclinations, and nutritional needs.

By adhering to these nutritional guidelines supported by scientific evidence, individuals diagnosed with non-alcoholic fatty liver disease (NAFLD) can enable themselves to make well-informed dietary decisions and proactively enhance their liver health and overall quality of life.

CHAPTER TWO

A Balanced Plate Contributes To Liver Health

To promote liver health, it is essential to maintain a balanced plate by including nutrient-dense foods it and limiting refined foods, harmful lipids, and added carbohydrates. An ordinary balanced plate generally comprises:

1. Strive to adorn fifty percent of your plate with an assortment of vibrant vegetables and fruits. The fiber, vitamins, minerals, and antioxidants found in abundance in these foods can aid in inflammation reduction and promote healthy liver function.

2. Opt for whole grains over refined grains; brown rice, quinoa, cereals, and whole wheat bread are examples of such grains. Whole cereals aid in blood sugar regulation and promote satiety by providing fiber and vital nutrients.

3. Lean proteins are crucial for promoting liver health and should be incorporated into one's diet.

Lean protein sources, including fish, lean poultry, legumes, tofu, and tempeh, should be prioritized. These proteins have a reduced saturated fat content and may aid in the prevention of additional hepatic fat accumulation.

4. Incorporate into your dietary intake sources of healthful lipids, such as avocados, almonds, seeds, and olive oil. Omega-3 fatty acids and monounsaturated fats, which support heart and liver health and have anti-inflammatory properties, are found in these fats.

5. Restrict Intake of Added Sugars and Processed Foods: Adhere to a reduced intake of sweetened beverages, processed munchies, desserts, and foods that are rich in saturated fats and trans fats. These substances may exacerbate symptoms of NAFLD and prolong liver inflammation.

6. It is crucial to exercise portion control to avoid excess, which has the potential to induce weight gain and worsen the deposition of fat in the liver. Practice

mindful dining and utilize smaller dishes to savor each morsel and identify feelings of satiety.

7. Hydration: Ensure proper hydration by consuming copious amounts of water daily. Adequate hydration aids in the elimination of impurities from the body and supports liver function.

By assembling a nutrient-dense plate that is well-balanced, individuals with NAFLD can improve their weight management, liver health, and overall well-being.

Consuming Lean Proteins As Part Of Your Diet

Lean protein consumption is essential for individuals with NAFLD to maintain liver health and aid in weight management. Lean proteins supply metabolic function, muscle growth, and tissue repair with vital amino acids without contributing an excessive amount of saturated fat or calories. Incorporating lean proteins into your diet is as follows:

1. Select Skinless Poultry: For lean sources of protein, choose skinless poultry and turkey breasts. Reduce the saturated fat content by removing the epidermis before heating.

2. Incorporate Fatty Fish: Salmon, mackerel, trout, and sardines are examples of fatty fish that are abundant in omega-3 fatty acids, which support liver health and have anti-inflammatory properties. Aim to consume fatty fish no less than twice per week.

3. Incorporate Legumes and Beans: Legumes, including kidney beans, lentils, chickpeas, and black beans, are exceptional sources of fiber and protein derived from plants. Soups, salads, stews, and vegetarian dishes can benefit from the added protein and nutrients provided by legumes.

4. Consider Incorporating Tempeh and Tofu: These soy-based protein sources are adaptable and simple to integrate into a variety of recipes. Tempeh and tofu should be marinated in flavorful seasonings and condiments before grilling, roasting, or stir-frying.

5. Consume Nuts and Seeds as a Snack Nuts and seeds are nutrient-dense foods that are abundant in vitamins, minerals, protein, and healthy lipids. Nuts and seeds include almonds, hazelnuts, chia seeds, and pumpkin seeds. Snack between meals on a scattering of almonds or seeds for a gratifying experience.

6. Incorporate Dairy Products: For an excellent source of protein and calcium, select low-fat or fat-free dairy products, such as Greek yogurt, cottage cheese, and skim milk. Dairy products can be incorporated into smoothies, baked pastries, or consumed on their own.

7. Consider culinary Methods: To preserve the nutritional value of lean proteins, choose healthy culinary methods such as grilling, roasting, simmering, and sautéing with minimal oil.

In addition to managing NAFLD symptoms, consuming lean proteins can support liver health, preserve muscle mass, and promote general well-being.

Vital Fats To Promote Liver Health

The consumption of healthful lipids is particularly crucial for individuals with NAFLD to maintain liver health and overall well-being. Antioxidants, fat-soluble vitamins, and essential fatty acids found in healthy lipids are responsible for nutrient assimilation, hormone production, and cell membrane functionality. The following are some dietary sources of healthful lipids to consider:

1. Avocados are an excellent source of monounsaturated lipids, specifically oleic acid, which has been scientifically demonstrated to enhance liver health and reduce inflammation. Incorporate avocado slices into smoothies, salads, or sandwiches to impart a velvety consistency and heart-healthy lipids.

2. Nuts and Seeds: Almonds, walnuts, flaxseeds, chia seeds, and hemp seeds are rich in vitamin E,

alpha-linolenic acid (ALA), and omega-3 fatty acids. Nuts and seeds, when sprinkled on yogurt, oatmeal, or salads, contribute nutritional value and texture.

3. Olive Oil: Constant in Mediterranean cuisine, extra virgin olive oil is renowned for its antioxidants and high concentration of monounsaturated lipids. Incorporate olive oil into mild sautéing, salad dressings, sauces, and marinades to impart flavor and support hepatic well-being.

4. Salmon, mackerel, trout, and sardines are oily fish that are abundant in omega-3 fatty acids, EPA, and DHA, all of which support liver function and have anti-inflammatory properties. At least twice per week, incorporate fatty fish into your diet for maximum health benefits.

5. Coconut oil, despite its high saturated fat content, is known to contain medium-chain triglycerides (MCTs), which undergo distinct metabolic pathways within the body and potentially promote liver health.

When cooking or baking, use coconut oil sparingly to impart flavor and richness.

6. Seaweed and algae, including nori, spirulina, and chlorella, are considered to be nutrient-dense foods due to their substantial content of antioxidants, vitamins, minerals, and essential fatty acids. For a nutritional boost, incorporate seaweed and algae into soups, salads, sushi, and smoothies.

7. Dark Chocolate: Rich in flavonoids, polyphenols, and healthful lipids, dark chocolate with a high cocoa content has been shown to enhance liver function and reduce inflammation. Incorporate dark chocolate into a balanced diet in moderation.

For individuals with NAFLD, incorporating these sources of healthful lipids into their diet can promote overall well-being, reduce inflammation, and support liver health. Opt for whole food sources of healthy lipids and exercise portion control for maximum nutritional benefits.

In summary, the integration of lean proteins, the consumption of healthy lipids, and the construction of a well-balanced plate are fundamental elements of a cookbook designed to promote liver health and holistic wellness in individuals with NAFLD. Individuals with NAFLD can improve their quality of life, control symptoms, and impede the progression of the disease by incorporating nourishing food selections into their diets and establishing balanced eating routines.

Making Intelligent Choices Regarding Carbohydrates And Fiber

Dietary modifications play a critical role in the management of Non-Alcoholic Fatty Liver Disease (NAFLD), and it is essential to comprehend the significance of carbohydrates and fiber in this regard.

To impede the progression of NAFLD, which is characterized by excessive fat deposition in the liver, a balanced diet is required. A NAFLD cookbook emphasizes the importance of consuming carbohydrates and fiber prudently.

Although carbohydrates are the principal source of energy for the body, they are not all created equal. The blood sugar-raising effects of simple carbohydrates, which are present in refined cereals and saccharine foods, exacerbate the symptoms of NAFLD. On the other hand, complex carbohydrates, which are commonly found in whole grains, fruits, and vegetables, provide essential nutrients and sustained energy release, rendering them advantageous options for individuals with NAFLD.

A form of carbohydrate, fiber, is crucial in the management of NAFLD. It promotes satiety, facilitates digestion, and controls blood sugar levels. Certain fruits, legumes, and oats contain soluble fiber, which forms a gel-like substance when dissolved in water; this fiber aids in the regulation of blood glucose and cholesterol levels.

Viscous insoluble fiber, which is found in abundance in whole cereals and vegetables, promotes regular digestive movements and aids in the detoxification process, both of which are vital for the health of the liver.

A cookbook for individuals with NAFLD includes an assortment of complex carbohydrate, high-fiber recipes that promote liver health and function. Promoting the consumption of whole grains, including barley, quinoa, and brown rice, in conjunction with a diverse assortment of vibrant fruits and vegetables, guarantees a diet that is abundant in vital vitamins and minerals and nutrient-dense.

By prioritizing fiber-rich foods and making intelligent carbohydrate selections, individuals with NAFLD can effectively manage their condition and enhance their overall health.

The Significance Of Vitamins And Minerals In Liver Health

Due to the critical importance of vitamins and minerals in liver health, their incorporation into a NAFLD cookbook is essential for the effective management of this condition. Non-alcoholic fatty liver disease (NAFLD) is significantly correlated with suboptimal nutrient consumption and poor dietary decisions. By giving precedence to vital vitamins and minerals, individuals can promote hepatic function and slow the progression of NAFLD.

As a potent antioxidant, vitamin E counteracts oxidative stress and inflammation, both of which are prevalent in NAFLD. A conspicuous inclusion of vitamin E-rich foods, including almonds, spinach, and sunflower seeds, is recommended for a NAFLD cookbook. In patients with NAFLD, supplementation with vitamin E has demonstrated encouraging outcomes in terms of diminishing liver fat accumulation and enhancing liver enzyme levels.

Vitamin D, which is essential for liver health and has immunomodulatory properties, is another vital nutrient. Low levels of vitamin D are associated with the severity of NAFLD. The consumption of vitamin D-rich foods, such as fatty salmon, fortified dairy products, and eggs, may aid in the maintenance of optimal vitamin D levels and potentially mitigate the symptoms associated with NAFLD.

Additionally, minerals such as magnesium and zinc are vital to liver function. NAFLD patients frequently experience zinc deficiency, which is correlated with fibrosis and inflammation of the liver. Zinc is found in legumes, grains, and lean proteins. Magnesium, which is present in whole cereals, legumes, and verdant greens, supports glucose metabolism and insulin sensitivity, both of which are critical for the management of NAFLD.

Recipes that feature an assortment of vitamin and mineral-rich components should be prioritized in a cookbook for patients with NAFLD to promote liver health and combat the nutrient deficiencies that are frequently observed. By prioritizing nutrient-dense foods, individuals can optimize their dietary consumption and bolster liver function, thereby augmenting their quality of life in its entirety.

CHAPTER THREE

The Effects Of Hydration On NAFLD: An Emphasis In The NAFLD Cookbook

Hydration is an essential component in the preservation of general well-being, encompassing hepatic functionality. In the context of non-alcoholic fatty liver disease (NAFLD), its importance cannot be exaggerated. NAFLD, being one of the most prevalent chronic liver diseases worldwide, requires substantial adjustments to one's lifestyle, with adequate hydration serving as a fundamental component.

Water is a fundamental component in numerous physiological processes, such as the detoxification of the liver and metabolic activities. Sufficient hydration promotes optimal hepatic blood flow, which in turn aids in the elimination of metabolic metabolites and pollutants. Moreover, adequate hydration promotes bile production, which facilitates the digestion and assimilation of fats—vital factors in the management of NAFLD.

By integrating hydrating foods, such as fruits and vegetables that are rich in water, into a cookbook for individuals with non-alcoholic fatty liver disease (NAFLD), one can effectively fulfill their daily fluid needs while also obtaining vital nutrients, minerals, and antioxidants. Cucumber, watermelon, celery, and citrus are all excellent examples of hydrating ingredients that can be incorporated into recipes that are NAFLD-friendly.

It is crucial to acknowledge that although water serves as the principal hydration source, additional fluid ingestion can be derived from medicinal infusions and coconut water, among others. However, individuals should restrict or abstain from consuming caffeinated beverages and alcohol, as these substances may worsen symptoms of NAFLD and contribute to hepatic damage.

Promoting proper hydration as an integral component of a comprehensive strategy for managing non-alcoholic fatty liver disease (NAFLD) enables individuals to proactively enhance their liver health and general state of being. By endorsing hydration-conscious practices via a NAFLD cookbook, individuals can enhance the efficacy of their dietary selections and facilitate their progress towards liver and lifestyle health.

Methods Of Meal Planning For NAFLD:

The management of NAFLD is significantly influenced by meal planning, which empowers patients to make informed dietary decisions that promote liver health and maintain a well-balanced intake. The following are some efficacious approaches delineated in NAFLD cookbooks:

1. NAFLD cookbooks place significant emphasis on the consumption of whole, unadulterated foods that are abundant in antioxidants and nutrients. Fruits, vegetables, lean proteins, whole cereals, nuts, seeds,

and legumes are all examples. In addition to offering vital vitamins, minerals, and fiber, whole foods help individuals decrease their consumption of refined carbohydrates, harmful lipids, and added sugars.

2. Saturated and trans fats exacerbate NAFLD and contribute to inflammation in the liver. Limit your intake of these unhealthy fats. Instead of these fats, cookbook recommendations frequently propose substituting them with more healthful substitutes, including monounsaturated and polyunsaturated fats that are present in avocado, olive oil, almonds, and oily fish such as salmon and mackerel.

3. Adherence to Portion Control: Effective portion control is critical for weight management and the prevention of excessive caloric consumption, both of which can exacerbate non-alcoholic fatty liver disease (NAFLD). In addition to providing guidance on suitable portion sizes for different food categories, cookbooks also endorse mindful eating strategies that encourage feeling full and discourage excessive consumption.

4. Utilize Liver-Cleansing Ingredients: Specific food items contain hepatoprotective properties that facilitate the process of liver detoxification. The incorporation of antioxidant and anti-inflammatory properties-associated ingredients such as turmeric, garlic, ginger, cruciferous vegetables, green tea, and citrus fruits is recommended in NAFLD cookbooks.

5. Maintain sufficient hydration to support optimal liver function and overall well-being. It is advised by NAFLD manuals to consume copious amounts of water daily, choose hydrating beverages such as herbal teas, infused water, and coconut water, and limit the consumption of sweetened sodas and fruit juices.

Through the adoption of these meal planning strategies, individuals diagnosed with NAFLD can efficiently enhance their dietary practices and effectively foster liver health.

Recipes For Delectable And Liver-Friendly Breakfasts:

A hearty brunch establishes a favorable atmosphere for the day and has the potential to greatly influence the health of the liver. The following brunch preparations, which are liver-friendly, are featured in NAFLD cookbooks:

1. Spinach and Avocado Omelette:

Combine the eggs and a dash of milk in a whisk.

- Stir in the minced spinach and diced avocado.

- Cook until set in a nonstick skillet.

- Complement with freshly harvested fruit as an accompaniment to enhance the antioxidant content.

2. Pureed chia seeds overnight:

- Incorporate a pinch of vanilla extract and unsweetened almond milk into the chia seeds.

Refrigerate until thickened, overnight.

- For added flavor, garnish with sliced almonds, diced mango, and a drizzle of honey.

3. Whole Grain Bowl for Breakfast:

- Prepare steel-cut quinoa or oats per the instructions on the package.

- Sprinkle with cinnamon, sliced bananas, and hazelnuts before topping with Greek yogurt.

To impart an organic sweetness, drizzle with one teaspoon of honey.

These breakfast recipes are rich in vital vitamins and minerals, nutrient-dense, and fiber-rich substances that promote overall health and liver function.

Ideas For Nutrient-Dense Lunches For NAFLD

Lunch is a time to incorporate palatable and gratifying options that additionally support liver health while providing an opportunity to incorporate nutrients into the diet.

The following are some suggestions for preparing nutritious meals for those who are managing NAFLD:

1. Salmon Salad with Avocado: Omega-3 fatty acids, which are present in salmon, have been shown to promote liver health and inflammation reduction. Slices of avocado, mixed vegetables, cherry tomatoes, and cucumber should be combined with seared or roasted salmon. For enhanced flavor, garnish with a delicate vinaigrette composed of olive oil and lemon juice.

2. Quinoa and Vegetable Stir-fry: A protein-rich and nutrient-dense whole grain, quinoa is an outstanding selection for those with non-alcoholic fatty liver disease (NAFLD). Incorporate a variety of vibrant vegetables, including bell peppers, broccoli, carrots, and snap peas, while stir-frying prepared quinoa. Incorporate lean protein sources such as grilled chicken or tofu into a well-balanced meal.

3. Consider utilizing whole-grain tortillas that are stuffed with hummus, spinach leaves, sliced cucumbers, and lean turkey breast.

Turkey is an exemplary source of protein that is low in saturated fat, whereas hummus contributes flavor and advantageous nutrients such as fiber and antioxidants.

4. Soups containing an abundance of vegetables and legumes, such as lentils, provide a nourishing and comforting meal. A substantial vegetable and lentil broth can be prepared by combining an assortment of vegetables, including carrots, celery, onions, and spinach. Herbs and seasonings such as cumin and turmeric impart additional anti-inflammatory properties.

5. Quinoa salad featuring legumes, diced bell peppers, red scallions, fresh herbs, and a piquant lemon-tahini vinaigrette should be assembled.

In contrast to quinoa, which is a complete source of essential amino acids and plant-based protein, chickpeas contain fiber.

By integrating these nourishing lunch suggestions into a diet that is compatible with NAFLD, one can promote liver health and overall vitality.

CHAPTER FOUR

Appetizing Dishes To Promote Liver Health:

1. Salmon grilled alongside steamed vegetables and quinoa:

Salmon, being abundant in omega-3 fatty acids, is a nutritional resource that aids in inflammation reduction and hepatic health promotion.

• Quinoa: An excellent source of complex carbohydrates rich in fiber, quinoa assists digestion and regulates blood sugar, thereby decreasing the risk of fatty liver disease.

• Steamed vegetables: Broccoli, asparagus, and Brussels sprouts are commendable selections, as they are rich in minerals, vitamins, and antioxidants that aid in the detoxification pathways of the liver.

2. Soup made with lentils and whole grain bread:

Legumes, which are rich in protein and fiber, promote satiety and aid in blood sugar regulation, making them an excellent food option for those with NAFLD.

• Whole grain bread is an excellent source of sustained energy and digestive health support due to its high fiber and complex carbohydrate content.

A vegetable broth base not only contributes to the dish's flavor but also maintains its minimal saturated fat and sodium content, both of which are essential for maintaining liver health.

3. Stir-fried turkey and Vegetables with Brown Rice:

• Lean turkey, being a lean protein source, possesses vital amino acids that are indispensable for liver repair and regeneration while also being low in saturated lipids.

• Vivid Vegetables: Snap peas, carrots, and bell peppers contribute zest and an assortment of essential nutrients, such as vitamins A and C, which are critical for the process of liver detoxification.

Brown rice, being a complex carbohydrate characterized by a low glycemic index, facilitates weight management, which is a critical aspect in the regulation of non-alcoholic fatty liver disease (NAFLD).

4. Chicken breast baked with spinach and sweet potato salad:

• Chicken Breast: A staple in liver-friendly diets, chicken breast is lean and protein-rich, providing essential nutrients without superfluous lipids.

• Sweet potato: Boasting a high content of fiber, vitamins, and antioxidants, sweet potatoes support liver function by regulating blood sugar levels and reducing inflammation.

Spinach salad, enhanced with a delicate vinaigrette dressing, contributes to liver detoxification and overall health through its high iron, folate, and vitamin K content.

Snack Alternatives That Promote Liver Function

The impact of snacks on liver health is contingent upon the selections made. Individuals diagnosed with NAFLD must select refreshments that are nutritious, low in saturated lipids and refined sugars, and low in saturated fat. The following snacks are beneficial to liver function:

1. Nuts such as pistachios, almonds, and walnuts are abundant in antioxidants, fiber, and healthful lipids. The reduction of inflammation and enhancement of insulin sensitivity are both advantageous in the context of NAFLD.

2. Greek Yogurt with Berries: Probiotics and protein, both of which aid digestion and promote digestive health, are abundant in Greek yogurt. Strawberries, blueberries, and raspberries are rich in antioxidants, vitamins, and minerals and are low in sugar.

3. Vegetable sticks accompanied by hummus, such as carrots, celery, and bell peppers, constitute a gratifying and nourishing refreshment option. In contrast to the protein and healthful lipids found in hummus, vegetables provide vital vitamins and minerals.

4. Avocado Toast: The fruit avocado is an excellent source of fiber, numerous vitamins and minerals, and nutrient-dense monounsaturated lipids. The fiber and complex carbohydrates found in whole-grain bread elevate avocado toast to the status of a well-balanced sustenance option.

5. A handcrafted trail mix, composed of a combination of nuts, seeds, and dried fruits, offers a gratifying refreshment that is additionally enriched with antioxidants, healthy lipids, and fiber. Raw almonds and unadulterated desiccated fruits are healthier alternatives for reducing the intake of added sugars and toxic lipids.

A Variation On Desserts: Delightful Treats For NAFLD

Managing NAFLD while satisfying a chocolate tooth can be difficult, but not insurmountable. Desserts can be enhanced in terms of taste and liver health by integrating nutritious components and making considered substitutions:

1. Fruit Salad with Mint: An invigorating fruit salad composed of an assortment of fruits including kiwi, watermelon, and pineapple, enhanced with a delicate sheen of honey and adorned with fresh mint, presents an ecologically sound and nourishing alternative to a dessert.

2. Chia seed pudding contains antioxidants, omega-3 fatty acids, and fiber in abundance. Unsweetened almond milk, chia seeds, vanilla extract, and a natural sweetener such as stevia or maple syrup are combined to produce a velvety and scrumptious custard that does not contain any added carbohydrates.

3. Baked Apples with Cinnamon: A decadent and guilt-free confection, baked apples dusted with cinnamon and drizzled with honey or maple syrup. In addition to their high fiber and antioxidant content, apples may also assist in enhancing insulin sensitivity.

4. Frozen Yogurt Bark is a delectable and customizable frozen delight made from Greek yogurt, a dash of pure vanilla extract, and a baking sheet. It is decorated with dark chocolate pieces, almonds, and seeds, and then frozen until firm.

5. Coconut Mango Sorbet: Freeze frozen mango segments until firm, then blend with coconut milk and a squeeze of lime juice. Comprised of antioxidants, minerals, and vitamins, this sorbet devoid of dairy provides a revitalizing and fortifying alternative to a dessert.

Liquids Influencing Liver Health

1. Sufficient hydration facilitates optimal metabolic function and aids in the detoxification processes of the liver, thereby supporting its operation. The predominant beverage selection in the NAFLD diet should be water.

2. Herbal Teas: Specific types of herbal teas, including dandelion root tea and green tea, are known to contain antioxidant properties that have the potential to mitigate liver inflammation and enhance liver health. They may serve as superior substitutes for caffeinated or sweetened beverages.

3. Vegetable juices that have been recently extracted, especially those that comprise liver-beneficial components such as beets, carrots, kale, and spinach, have the potential to supply the liver with a concentrated supply of antioxidants and nutrients that aid in its functioning.

4. Smoothies: Individuals with NAFLD may find nutrient-dense smoothies containing verdant greens,

berries, avocado, and flaxseeds to be hydrating and nourishing.

5. Alcohol Substitutes with Limitations: Although individuals with NAFLD should abstain from consuming alcoholic beverages, certain non-alcoholic alternatives such as mocktails or alcohol-free beer can provide a social alternative devoid of the detrimental impacts that alcohol has on the liver.

CHAPTER FIVE

Practices Of Mindful Eating For NAFLD:

1. Mindful eating incorporates portion control by directing attention towards signals of appetite and satiety, decelerating during meals, and valuing every mouthful. To effectively manage NAFLD, portion control is essential, as excessive caloric intake, even from nutritious foods, can contribute to the accumulation of liver fat and metabolic dysfunction.

2. Balanced Meals: The NAFLD cookbook advocates for the consumption of well-balanced meals, which comprise an assortment of nutritious lipids, lean proteins, complex carbohydrates, fruits, and vegetables. This equilibrium influences insulin sensitivity and blood sugar regulation, both of which are crucial for the management of NAFLD.

3. Meal Planning and Preparation: Individuals with non-alcoholic fatty liver disease (NAFLD) can exert greater control over their dietary intake by

organizing meals in advance and preparing homemade dishes with fresh, whole ingredients. This ensures that they consume foods that promote liver health while avoiding those that may worsen the condition.

4. Engaging in mindful snacking entails selecting foods that are rich in nutrients, such as fresh produce, almonds, yogurt, or vegetable skewers accompanied by humus. Preventing aimless nibbling on manufactured foods that are loaded with harmful lipids and sugar aids in the regulation of blood sugar levels and promotes the overall health of the liver.

5. Stress Management: In addition to promoting improper dietary behaviors and inciting inflammation in the body, stress can exacerbate NAFLD. To promote relaxation and general well-being, mindful dining practices incorporate stress-relieving techniques such as deep breathing, meditation, and engaging in pleasurable activities.

A Comprehension Of Portion Control

A fundamental component of managing NAFLD and promoting overall health is portion control. It entails controlling the portion sizes of food consumed during meals and snacks to prevent excessive eating and sustain healthy body weight. The following are some techniques for implementing portion control:

1. Utilize Visual Cues: Individuals can assist in determining appropriate serving sizes by utilizing visual cues, such as portion control dishes or comparing food portions to commonplace objects (e.g., a deck of cards for meat).

2. By consulting food labels, individuals can enhance their ability to regulate their caloric intake and make well-informed decisions regarding portion control by familiarizing themselves with the serving sizes indicated.

3. Engage in Mindful consuming: By attending to signals of hunger and satiety, consuming gradually,

and deriving pleasure from every mouthful, one can mitigate the risk of excess and increase contentment with reduced serving sizes.

4. Selecting smaller plates and dishes can deceive the mind into believing that smaller portions are sufficient, thereby decreasing the probability of excess.

5. Pre-portion foods: Individuals can better adhere to portion sizes and prevent aimless snacking by dividing foods into single-serving portions in advance.

In summary, the NAFLD cookbook provides informative recommendations regarding the choice of beverages that promote hepatic health, the implementation of mindful eating strategies, and the mastery of portion control to efficiently handle NAFLD and enhance general health. By integrating these principles into their daily dietary routines, individuals diagnosed with non-alcoholic fatty liver disease (NAFLD) can proactively mitigate the risk of disease progression and enhance liver function.

A Knowledge Of NAFLD-Compatible Cooking Methods

Achieving a NAFLD-friendly cookbook necessitates the incorporation of cookery methodologies that not only safeguard liver health but also guarantee palatable and gratifying fare. Listed below are some crucial techniques:

1. Baking and Grilling: Because baking and grilling contain fewer added lipids than frying, they assist in regulating caloric consumption and restricting saturated and trans fats, which can both exacerbate non-alcoholic fatty liver disease (NAFLD).

2. Boiling and steaming are both effective methods for preparing lean proteins and vegetables. They aid in nutrient retention and eliminate the requirement for excessive lipids or oils.

3. Substitute healthful lipids for saturated and trans fats in your diet, such as almonds, olive oil, and

avocado oil. These lipids are advantageous for cardiovascular health and may aid in the reduction of hepatic inflammation.

4. Portion Control: To effectively manage NAFLD, portion control is vital. Appropriate portion sizes should be emphasized in NAFLD cookbooks to discourage overloading and excessive caloric consumption.

5. Achieving Balanced Meals: Organize your meals in a balanced fashion by incorporating an abundance of fruits and vegetables, lean proteins, whole cereals, and healthy lipids. By adopting a balanced approach, individuals can effectively manage their weight and liver health while ensuring they receive vital nutrients.

Integrating Physical Activity Into One's Daily Routine

Physical activity is essential for the management of NAFLD. Consistent physical activity enhances insulin sensitivity, diminishes hepatic adiposity, and advances general health and welfare. Listed below are some suggestions for making physical activity a part of your daily life:

1. Select Pleasurable Activities: Whether it be dancing, swimming, walking, or cycling, opt for activities that please you, as this will increase the likelihood that you will maintain them consistently.

2. Commence Activity Gradually and Elevate Intensity: In the case of individuals who are inactive or new to exercise, commence with low-intensity exercises and progressively augment both the duration and intensity of the routine as their fitness level advances.

3. Engage in Physical Activity with a Companion: Having a family member or companion accompany you on your workouts can increase your motivation and hold you accountable.

4. Establish a Routine: Incorporate consistent exercise sessions into your weekly timetable, analogous to how you would approach any other

scheduled appointment. Consistency is critical for achieving success.

5. Diversify Your Efforts: Protect against tedium by integrating a variety of activities into your daily schedule. Diverse your exercise regimen to include flexibility exercises, strength training, and cardiovascular activities.

6. Observe your body's sensations both during and following physical activity. In the event of encountering pain or discomfort, modify your daily regimen accordingly and, if required, seek the guidance of a healthcare professional.

Techniques For Managing Stress To Promote Liver Health

By inducing unhealthy coping mechanisms, such as gorging or the consumption of high-fat comfort foods, stress can worsen NAFLD. Consequently, techniques for stress management are essential for promoting liver health. The following are several efficacious strategies:

1. Meditation and Mindfulness: Engaging in meditation and mindfulness practices can aid in tension reduction and relaxation. Dedicate a few minutes daily to engage in guided meditation or deep breathing exercises.

2. Yoga and Tai Chi are forms of low-intensity physical activity that integrate mindfulness and breathing techniques. They have the potential to alleviate tension and enhance general welfare.

3. Consistent Physical Activity: In addition to promoting physical well-being, consistent physical activity aids in stress reduction and mood enhancement through the secretion of endorphins, which are endogenous stress relievers within the body.

4. Adopting healthy lifestyle practices, including maintaining adequate sleep, consuming a well-balanced diet, and refraining from excessive alcohol and caffeine intake, can aid in stress reduction and liver health promotion.

5. It is advisable to promptly seek support from family members, acquaintances, or a mental health professional when faced with distressing situations. Communicating one's emotions and apprehensions can facilitate the reduction of tension and offer a feeling of solace.

In summary, the NAFLD Cookbook integrates culinary methods that are compatible with NAFLD, underscores the significance of engaging in physical activity, and provides stress management tactics as a means to enhance hepatic health. By incorporating these principles into one's daily routine, one can proficiently regulate NAFLD and enhance their holistic health.

CHAPTER SIX

Guidelines For Eating Away With NAFLD

Individuals with Non-Alcoholic Fatty Liver Disease (NAFLD) may encounter difficulties when dining out due to the prevalence of toxic lipids, carbohydrates, and sodium-rich dishes on restaurant menus. However, by exercising strategic forethought and making conscientious decisions, it is feasible to savor dining at restaurants while keeping liver health in mind. The following are suggestions for dining out with NAFLD:

1. Conduct Pre-dinner Research: Before dining out, allocate sufficient time to investigate local restaurants that provide menu options that are more conducive to good health. The availability of nutritional information on the websites of numerous restaurants enables patrons to make more informed decisions regarding their orders.

2. Select Dining Establishments with Healthier Choices: I seek out establishments that prioritize the use of fresh, whole ingredients and provide a menu that can be customized. Choose dining establishments that offer a variety of vegetable-based dishes, salads, and grilled or roasted proteins.

3. Consider Portion Sizes: Restaurant servings are typically more substantial in size compared to portions that one might prepare at home. To prevent excess, consider sharing an entree with a dining companion or requesting a half portion.

4. Request Modifications: To accommodate your dietary requirements, please do not hesitate to request modifications from your server. To reduce added lipids and carbohydrates, request steamed vegetables or a side salad instead of fries or potatoes, and request dressings and condiments on the side.

5. Fried and Greasy Foods to Avoid: Dishes that are excessively breaded and deep-fried should be avoided, as they are frequently high in unhealthy

lipids and calories. Select alternatives that are roasted, broiled, or grilled as they contain less cholesterol and are more beneficial for liver health.

6. Limit Alcohol Consumption: Alcoholic beverages can contribute to the progression of NAFLD and exacerbate liver inflammation. Consider low-alcohol or non-alcoholic alternatives, such as unsweetened iced tea or carbonated water with citrus.

7. Adherence to Portion Control Regarding Desserts: In the event of a sweet tooth, contemplate the option of sharing a dessert with the table or selecting a fruit-infused alternative such as sorbet or fresh berries. Exercise portion control and select delicacies that contain minimal amounts of saturated fats and added carbohydrates.

8. Observe Your Body's Reactions: Track the emotional impact of various cuisines and the physical manifestations that ensue from dining out. Observe any symptoms or discomfort that may arise,

and modify your dining selections accordingly for subsequent occasions.

9. Maintain Hydration: To ensure optimal liver function and to remain hydrated, consume copious amounts of water throughout your meal. Replace saccharine beverages with water, herbal tea, or carbonated water when seeking to rejuvenate oneself.

10. It is crucial to exercise moderation and enjoyment when dining. Although it is significant to be cognizant of one's dietary preferences, it is equally vital to appreciate the flavors and social interaction that accompany communal meals.

By implementing these recommendations and tactics, individuals diagnosed with NAFLD can effectively navigate the dining experience at restaurants while placing their liver health and general well-being first. By making informed and conscientious decisions, dining out can be a pleasurable experience that also contributes to the maintenance of a NAFLD-friendly diet.

Progress Monitoring And Commemorating Achievements

Managing NAFLD effectively requires dietary modifications in addition to progress surveillance and recognition of milestones reached. Monitoring one's progress allows for the evaluation of how dietary modifications affect the health of the liver and overall state of being. The monitoring of progress and commemoration of achievements are pivotal components in the management of NAFLD:

1. The utilization of a food diary facilitates the monitoring of an individual's dietary consumption, enabling the identification of possible triggers or patterns that could worsen symptoms associated with NAFLD. The act of documenting symptoms such as fatigue, abdominal distress, or fluctuations in energy levels enables individuals to establish a connection between these symptoms and their dietary decisions,

thereby promoting the implementation of well-informed modifications.

2. Consistent Medical Examinations and Assessments: It is critical to undergo routine medical examinations and liver function tests to monitor the advancement of NAFLD and evaluate the efficacy of dietary interventions. Continually monitoring insulin resistance, liver enzymes, and cholesterol levels yields invaluable information regarding liver health and metabolic function.

3. The management of NAFLD necessitates adherence to a healthy weight regimen, given that excessive weight is a contributing factor to the accumulation of liver fat and metabolic dysfunction. Consistently monitoring weight loss progress via weigh-ins enables individuals to maintain motivation and adapt their lifestyle choices and dietary practices accordingly.

4. Enhancements in Health Parameters and Biomarkers: Positive fluctuations in biomarkers,

including lipid profiles, blood glucose levels, and liver enzyme levels, serve as indicators of improved metabolic function and liver health. Commemorating declines in hepatic adiposity and enhancements in insulin sensitivity serves to underscore the criticality of adhering to a healthy diet and inspire individuals to persist in their pursuit of optimal well-being.

5. Establishing Practical Objectives and Commemorating Conquerors: Establishing practical dietary and lifestyle objectives fosters longevity and sustainability in the management of non-alcoholic fatty liver disease (NAFLD). Commemorating accomplishments, such as attaining a significant weight loss milestone, enhancing dietary practices, or decreasing hepatic fat content, serve to strengthen constructive behavior modifications and inspire people to sustain their endeavors.

6. Enhancing Variety and Satisfaction: By integrating a selection of nutrient-dense foods into the diet and attempting out new recipes, one can increase both enjoyment and adherence to dietary

recommendations. Indulging in delectable, liver-friendly fare to commemorate accomplishments entails providing nourishment to the body and promoting liver health.

7. Pursuing Encouragement and Support: Establishing a support network comprising healthcare professionals, family members, and colleagues offers valuable guidance and motivation during the course of managing non-alcoholic fatty liver disease (NAFLD). Engaging in collective celebrations of accomplishments cultivates a feeling of community and underscores the criticality of sustained assistance in attaining ideal health results.

In essence, monitoring advancements and commemorating achievements are fundamental elements in the management of NAFLD and the advancement of general health. Through the consistent monitoring of dietary and lifestyle modifications, individuals can efficiently regulate non-alcoholic fatty liver disease (NAFLD), enhance the health of their livers, and commemorate significant milestones in their journey toward wellness.

Frequent Concerns Regarding NAFLD And Diet

Complex in nature, Non-Alcoholic Fatty Liver Disease (NAFLD) is impacted by a multitude of factors, one of which is dietary intake. By providing answers to frequently asked questions regarding NAFLD and diet, individuals can enhance their comprehension of the correlation between dietary selections and liver health. This knowledge empowers them to make well-informed decisions and manage the condition more efficiently.

1. What is the significance of diet in the pathogenesis and treatment of NAFLD?

• A substantial role is played by diet in the development and management of NAFLD. A diet high in processed foods, refined carbohydrates, and saturated fats contributes to the accumulation of liver fat and metabolic dysfunction. Adopting a well-balanced diet that is abundant in whole cereals, fruits, vegetables, lean proteins, and healthy lipids reduces the risk of NAFLD progression and promotes liver health.

2. Do specific dietary recommendations exist for those who have been diagnosed with NAFLD?

• It is true that dietary guidelines for individuals diagnosed with non-alcoholic fatty liver disease (NAFLD) center around the following: calorie restriction, weight maintenance, and attainment, moderation of alcohol consumption, the inclusion of liver-friendly foods (e.g., leafy greens, fatty fish, nuts, seeds, and olive oil), and limitation of sugary beverages and foods rich in added sugars.

3. How can I include nutrients that are beneficial to the liver in my diet?

One can optimize their dietary intake of foods that are beneficial for the liver by organizing well-balanced meals that emphasize the use of ingredients rich in nutrients. A balanced diet that incorporates an assortment of fruits, vegetables, whole cereals, lean proteins, and healthy lipids supports liver function and metabolic health while ensuring adequate nutrient intake.

4. Should individuals with NAFLD refrain from consuming any particular nutrients or foods?

• Foods that are rich in added sugars, refined carbohydrates, saturated fats, and trans fats should be avoided or restricted by those with NAFLD, as these substances contribute to the accumulation of liver fat and inflammation. By reducing intake of processed foods, fast food, caffeinated treats, and fried foods, the risk of NAFLD progression can be mitigated.

5. Can nutritional supplements aid in the management of NAFLD?

Although dietary supplements can enhance the benefits of a healthy diet, their efficacy in the management of NAFLD is still uncertain. Specific dietary supplements, including milk thistle, omega-3 fatty acids, and vitamin E, have demonstrated promise in promoting liver health and decreasing hepatic lipid accumulation. Before integrating supplements into your regimen, it is imperative that you seek guidance from a healthcare professional due to the potential for interactions with medications or the occurrence of adverse effects.

6. How can I sustainably modify my diet to help manage NAFLD?

• To achieve sustainable dietary adjustments, one must modify food behaviors progressively, establish attainable objectives, and solicit assistance from registered dietitians, healthcare professionals, and support groups. Adopting a well-rounded and varied dietary regimen, engaging in consistent physical activity, and practicing mindful eating all contribute to sustaining compliance with dietary guidelines and bolstering the overall health of the liver.

By responding to frequently requested inquiries regarding NAFLD and diet, individuals acquire significant knowledge regarding dietary approaches to effectively manage the condition and enhance liver health. By providing individuals with information and direction, they can make well-informed dietary decisions, encourage positive lifestyle changes, and improve their overall health as they strive to manage non-alcoholic fatty liver disease (NAFLD).

Conclusion

In summary, the Non-Alcoholic Fatty Liver Disease (NAFLD) Cookbook serves as an indispensable manual for those who wish to effectively address this widespread ailment by promoting their health and overall well-being. In light of the growing international recognition of NAFLD as a substantial health issue, dietary interventions are emerging as crucial approaches to its prevention and management.

Using a comprehensive collection of recipes designed to promote liver health and address the root causes of NAFLD, this cookbook provides an extensive selection. Through the prioritization of nutrient-dense, whole foods and the reduction of processed ingredients, this resource enables readers to make well-informed decisions that foster liver health and holistic well-being.

Furthermore, the recipes in the cookbook are both scrumptious and nutritious, debunking the fallacy that a healthy diet must sacrifice flavor and gratification. Employing inventive culinary techniques and combining unorthodox ingredients, motivates people to adopt a varied and pleasurable dietary regimen that is in harmony with their well-being objectives.

Moreover, in addition to functioning as a compilation of recipes, the NAFLD Cookbook promotes a comprehensive outlook on health through the provision of insightful information regarding the nutritional principles that support liver health. By enlightening readers regarding the influence of dietary decisions on the advancement of NAFLD, it enables them to adopt proactive measures in pursuit of bettering their health outcomes.

The NAFLD Cookbook serves as a significant resource in the fight against this widespread liver condition, providing not only physical sustenance but also motivation for individuals endeavoring to regain authority over their well-being and energy.

THE END

Printed in the USA
CPSIA information can be obtained
at www.ICGtesting.com
LVHW020238190924
791519LV00021B/275